Caspian Banki

Lynne Banki

What Autism Means To Me

forward by Lynne Banki

afterward by Patricia Byrne

published by Lifelight Books
Sammamish, WA USA

PUBLISHER

Lifelight Books published September 2003

ACKNOWLEDGEMENTS

A special word of thanks to Caspian's friends and classmates for the use of their words and artwork.

DESIGN

created using Adobe Photoshop and Adobe InDesign

layout and design by Lynne Banki using Caspian's artwork with contributing illustrations by Damian (p. 6, 11, 18) and Lynne (p. 21)

ISBN 0-9743801-0-5
PCN (Library of Congress Ctrl No): 2003096525

Lifelight Books
Sammamish, WA USA

for ordering info, please access
www.lifelightbooks.com

For my little brother Damian

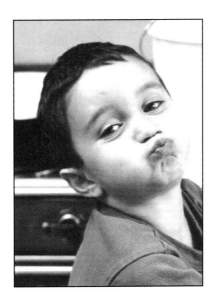

i love you

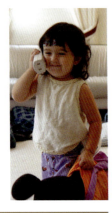
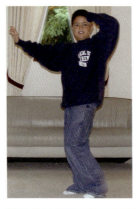
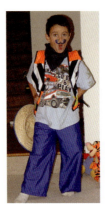

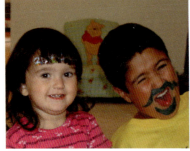
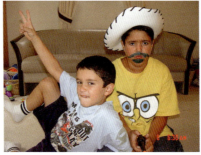
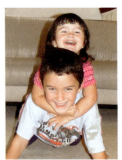

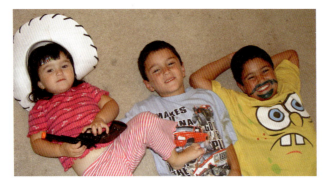
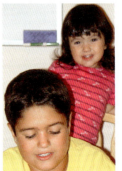

Family, move to the beat.
Family, mmm, that's sweet.
Family, while the world turns around
family keeps you safe and sound.
Jump, cross, turn around,
your family won't ever let you down!

from the song "Family Line Dance"
Happily Ever After
Songs by Howie McOmber

"Caspian, do you know what autism is?" I asked casually as we drove home from school. I couldn't believe I was doing this. "Yes," he replied, just a little too fast for me to be sure he had even heard the question. His 'yes' was perfect and studied. And no wonder. A few years ago it had taken me almost six months to teach him how to answer a question with the word yes. "What is it?" I pressed on. Questioning him in the car was always easiest. It required no eye contact. "I do not know", he said into space. I sighed quietly. I wasn't sure I wanted to do this.

Caspian was in his first few weeks of first grade when the teachers, his special needs coordinator, his part-time educational assistant and I sat down to marvel at his progress. I had braced myself for a tough start to the school year and was graced with just the opposite. Caspian's transition to full day could not have gone any better! He was happily going off to school and was not completely unreachable by the time his little brother Damian and I met him at the classroom door. No raging tantrums! I declared victory! Then his teachers shook my world. "Have you considered talking to the class about autism?" I whipped out a letter that I had prepared for the parents. Problem solved, I thought. "But what about his classmates? They're starting to notice some of his behavior." I froze. They couldn't be serious. Single him out? Already? I wasn't ready. We had worked so hard to get Caspian to this point. Why did the other kids need to know? He was doing so well! Wasn't he doing so well? "How can I tell his classmates that he's autistic? I haven't even told *him* yet!"

"Caspian, do you know what autistic is?" I remember the first time I told a perfect stranger that Caspian was autistic. We were in a grocery store and this kindly woman kept trying to talk with him. When she couldn't get his attention, she moved closer. He snapped out of his reverie just in time to see a big pair of shiny eyeglasses two inches from his nose. He screamed. She kept trying to make it right. She reached out to calm him. Her gentle touch made him arch his body so far back I thought he would fall into the back of the shopping cart. I frantically put my body between them. I really wanted to scream, "Get out of his face already, will you?" But instead I uttered, "It's not your fault, he's autistic." There, I had said it. I guess it was real. Over the years I had gotten better at intervening on his behalf. Cold shoulders and comments made under the breath were par for the course and no longer slicing. We've all been through it. There will always be those who blame parenting for neurology. Most people just don't understand what autism is. How it must appear to them when Caspian loses it; to this day we can still clear an aisle faster than a fire alarm!

I repeated the question. "Caspian, do you know what autistic is?" "Yes," he answered, matching his previous answer in both speed and tone. "What is it?" I tried again. Caspian took his thumbnail out of his mouth just long enough to answer. "A good kid."

Maybe this wasn't such a bad idea after all.

Lynne Banki (Caspian's mother)

Being autistic means

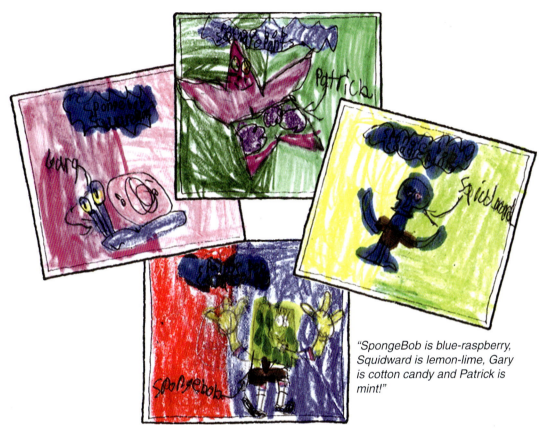

"SpongeBob is blue-raspberry, Squidward is lemon-lime, Gary is cotton candy and Patrick is mint!"

SpongeBob SquarePants Trading Cards

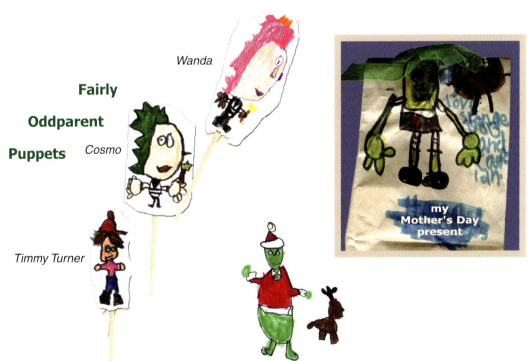

Fairly

Oddparent

Puppets

Wanda

Cosmo

Timmy Turner

my Mother's Day present

when I like something, I think about it all of the time. I used to play Grinch games a lot. Now I like anything to do with Nickelodeon!

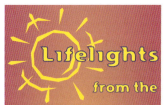

Lifelights from the SIDELINES

Every fixation, no matter how specific, can be used to hook and pull Caspian into new arenas.

Lynne (mother)

He cycles through movie favorites. Caspian has seen *The Lion King* so many times. He watches the video in all available languages, reads the book, and listens to different versions of the sound track.

Parviz (father)

SpongeBob fills his thoughts. Caspian often draws or uses SpongeBob in his work.

Ms. H (3rd grade teacher)

Two years ago I remember he gave out Grinch stories and coloring books. Now Caspian always talks about Nickelodeon!

Elise (classmate)

I remember when Caspian's mother asked me to make a Grinch costume for him. I thought the novelty would wear off quickly. A year or more later he was still finding reasons to wear the costume!

Jan (aunt)

He likes to talk about characters from his favorite shows. Sometimes he writes stories or creates games about them.

Anna (2nd & 3rd grade EA)

He always watches Nickelodeon.

Damian (brother)

When Caspian was little, he would carry around simple objects for weeks on end; like the block-shaped Sesame Street candles he held for so long they almost melted in his little fist. His attachments take on the form of thought now.

Lynne (mother)

We would notice this when holidays came around and we would forget to take an item away that had to do with a holiday. He would remind us that it was there until it disappeared (the Halloween pumpkin in the window).

Mrs. N (2nd grade teacher)

Being autistic means

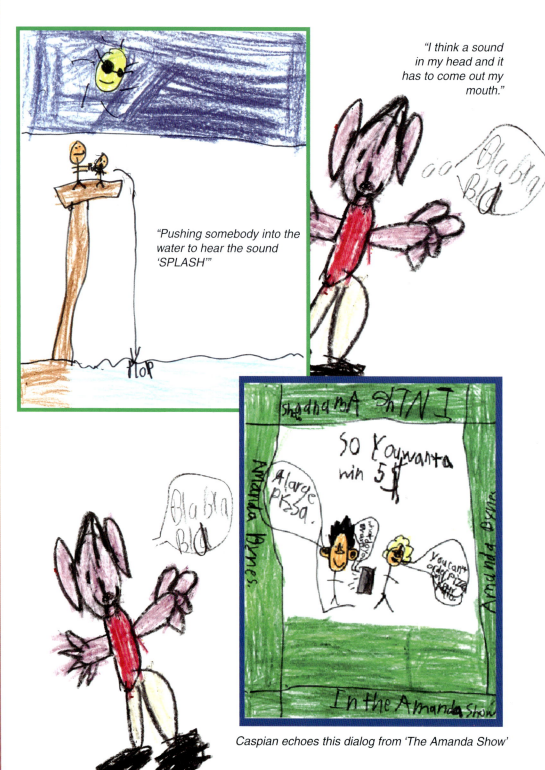

"I think a sound in my head and it has to come out my mouth."

"Pushing somebody into the water to hear the sound 'SPLASH'"

Caspian echoes this dialog from 'The Amanda Show'

words and sounds stick in my head. I like to say them or hear them over and over again. It makes me laugh!

Being autistic means

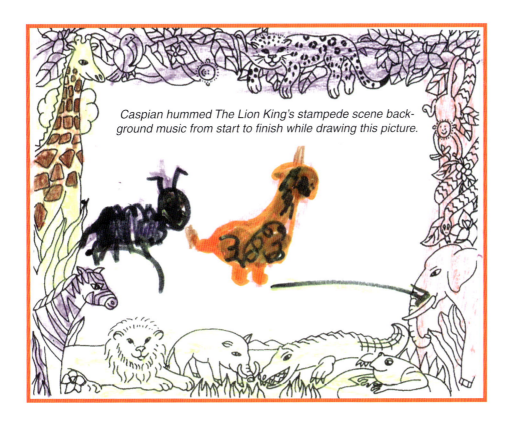

Caspian hummed The Lion King's stampede scene background music from start to finish while drawing this picture.

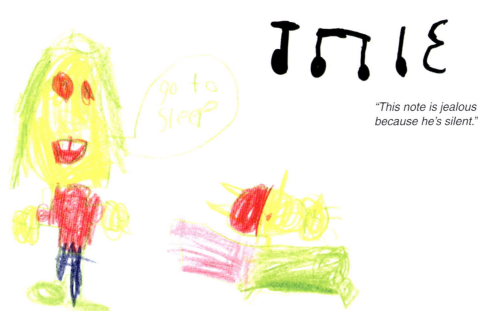

"This note is jealous because he's silent."

Slow songs, especially lullabies, would bring Caspian to tears. "I used to cry my sad out. Now it's OK. I just keep it inside."

I like music a lot, but slow songs make me very sad inside. I can remember almost every tune I hear and where I heard it first.

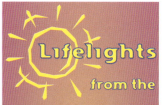

Lifelights
from the
SIDELINES

When I don't remember where a phrase or tune comes from, I ask Caspian. He *always* knows the answer.

Parviz (father)

He has been known to elaborate on a memory by humming what was playing in the background at the time. He is also amazing with theme recognition. Sound track subtleties are not wasted on him.

Lynne (mother)

A song changed; same music, new words. It was very disturbing to him.

Diane (2nd grade EA)

At the beginning of the year Caspian covered his ears at the singing of our school song.

Ms. H (3rd grade teacher)

He always sings the songs we learn in music class.

Elise (classmate)

I have heard Caspian analyze the differences in the same piece of music recorded by different people. Also he will point out the difference between the Broadway version and a movie sound track no matter how small. It's pretty amazing.

Jan (aunt)

Some songs make all of us sad sometimes. Such a great memory you have to be able to remember tunes and where you heard them first.

Joy (classroom volunteer)

He used to cry when he heard quiet music.

Damian (brother)

Prosody, the music of speech, became my ally. Once he understood *not now* spoken with a particular melody, I could expand his vocabulary by saying *maybe later* using the same pattern.

Lynne (mother)

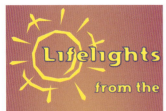

Being autistic means

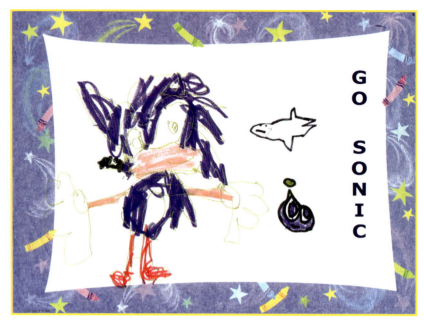

GO SONIC

SIDELINES

He is extremely visual and can literally see his way through a game. Internet searches showed him why spelling mattered. He is a great speller now.

Lynne (mother)

Whenever he gets stuck in a video game, he doesn't give up. He keeps going until he figures it out. For however many days it takes to complete the game, he lives it entirely.

Parviz (father)

Computers and video games are cut and dry. They don't give off opposite messages like people sometimes do.

Diane (2nd grade EA)

Caspian was able to make a Power Point presentation about rocks. He added effects and sounds by himself and was one of the first ones done. He was anxious to share his show with me.

Ms. H (3rd grade teacher)

He is always talking about Mario.

Elise (classmate)

Sometimes I play video games with Caspian and he always wins!

Jan (aunt)

Caspian will sometimes focus really hard on a video game and it is tough to try and get him to do something else.

Scott (mentor)

You will probably make a great computer programmer someday.

Joy (classroom volunteer)

Oh, yeah. He really likes that!

Damian (brother)

Once he figured out how the mouse worked, there was no stopping him. Getting him to figure out how the mouse worked was another story. He became motivated by the desire to hear his favorite theme song played over and over. He needed to click on the *play* button on screen, a shape and action he recognized from his toy tape player.

Lynne (mother)

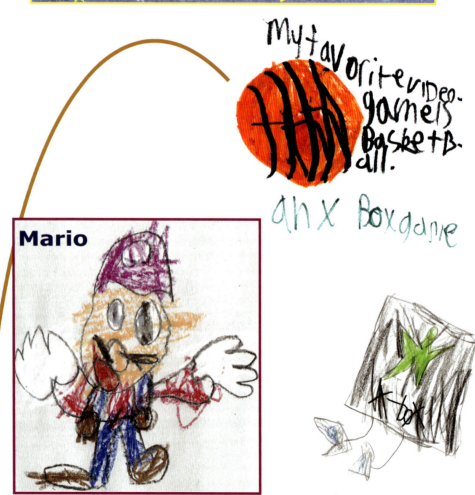

I am very good at video games and I really like computers.

4

What do you like?

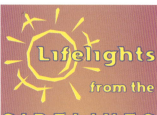

Being autistic means

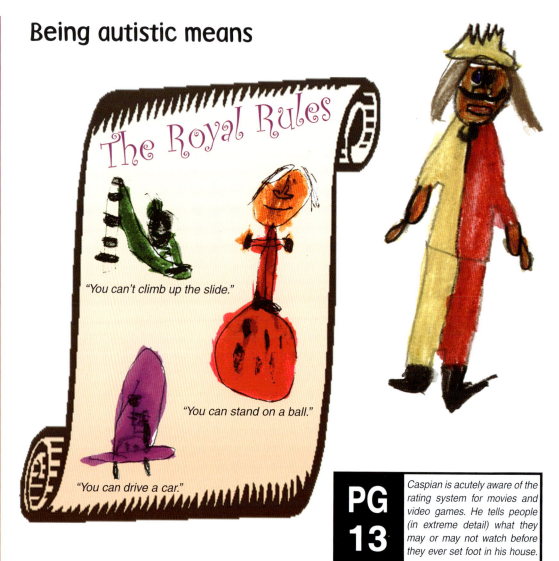

The Royal Rules

"You can't climb up the slide."

"You can stand on a ball."

"You can drive a car."

PG 13 Caspian is acutely aware of the rating system for movies and video games. He tells people (in extreme detail) what they may or may not watch before they ever set foot in his house.

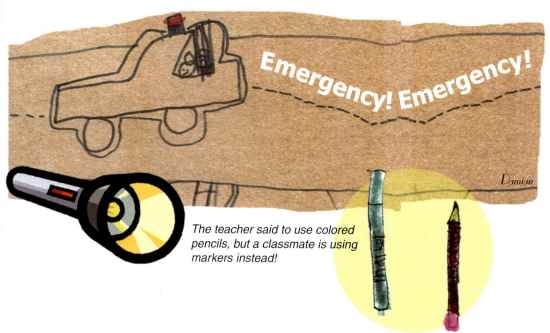

Emergency! Emergency!

Damian

The teacher said to use colored pencils, but a classmate is using markers instead!

I feel safe when people follow the rules, so I like to tell people what the rules are.

Being autistic means

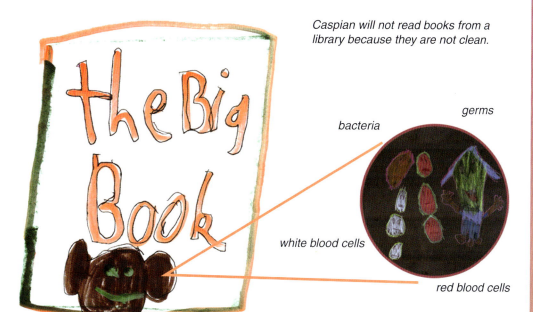

Caspian will not read books from a library because they are not clean.

germs

bacteria

white blood cells

red blood cells

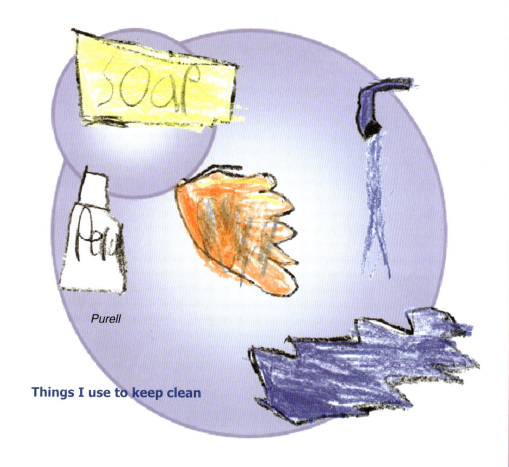

Purell

Things I use to keep clean

I feel safe when things are clean. Especially my hands!

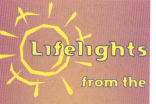
Caspian stopped playing in playgrounds for a long while because they were too dirty. Although he's since gotten over this, I still need to keep anti-bacterial gel accessible.

Lynne (mother)

He is constantly brushing his teeth.

Parviz (father)

A couple of times each morning I hear the water running in the back of the room and look up to see Caspian washing his hands. He rarely cleans the table and counter tops anymore.

Ms. H (3rd grade teacher)

Caspian always goes straight to the sink after art class to wash his hands

Rebecca (classmate)

Before lunch he always tells us to wash our hands.

Elise (classmate)

Germs are scary to him! Germs hurt people and make them sick or die. He can't see them, but he knows they are there.

Diane (2nd grade EA)

He has to take a shower after we play on the water slide.

Damian (brother)

I know this about Caspian. But I've seen both sides of it. He'll sneeze or cough and be ready to train again without thinking about how his germs might effect others.

Jennifer (martial arts instructor)

Before Caspian had a concept of clean and dirty, it was texture that bothered him most. He wouldn't touch anything that felt like foam, for example, yet he would play in the mud for hours. The light touch of wispy things like long hair on a stuffed animal frightened him, and for some time he would not touch or walk on patterned surfaces.

Lynne (mother)

What makes you feel safe and secure?

Being autistic means

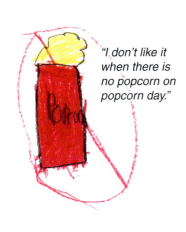

"I don't like it when there is no popcorn on popcorn day."

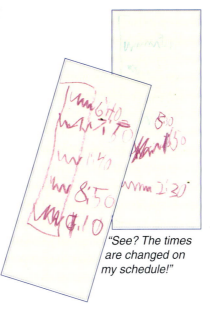

"See? The times are changed on my schedule!"

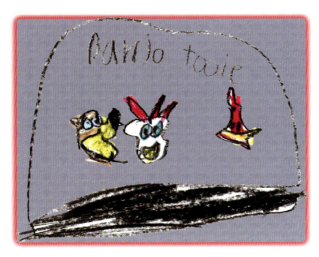

A rented video game and a newly-owned video game do **not** appear the same!
Missing (unearned) characters and levels cause confusion and rage.

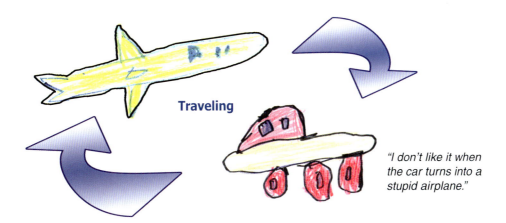

Traveling

"I don't like it when the car turns into a stupid airplane."

I don't feel calm when things are different. I feel most safe when things don't change.

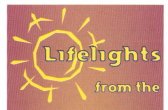

Lifelights from the SIDELINES

It doesn't matter how long things take as long as everything is in the right order.
Lynne (mother)

Caspian would rather stay home than do anything else. The simple things are a struggle. When we do go out, it can never be to someplace new.
Parviz (father)

If Caspian's schedule is going to change he likes you to tell him about it early so he can think about it for awhile. Unexpected changes make him uneasy.
Mr. G (1st grade teacher)

One time I was supposed to sleep over and I changed my mind. He cried for a long time. I felt really bad.
Alejandro (friend)

Caspian reads the daily schedule and always asks about changes. He persists until his questions and concerns are answered.
Ms. H (3rd grade teacher)

Caspian always stayed at the same desk in 2nd grade but now in third grade he gets to move.
Rebecca (classmate)

The teacher usually tells him where he is moving to or he just doesn't move.
Elise (classmate)

Things always change - even the weather. Caspian is getting much more flexible this year.
Joy (classroom volunteer)

We were supposed to go to the pool but then I got sick. Caspian got **very** disappointed.
Damian (brother)

When I visit, I break the routine. Sometimes this makes Caspian angry. I also need to make sure that I don't arrive after he has gone to sleep. Waking up to a new person in the house is too disturbing.
Mina (grandmother)

Caspian and I tend to do a lot of the same things when we are hanging out.
Scott (mentor)

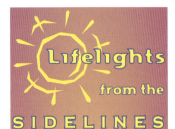

Being autistic means

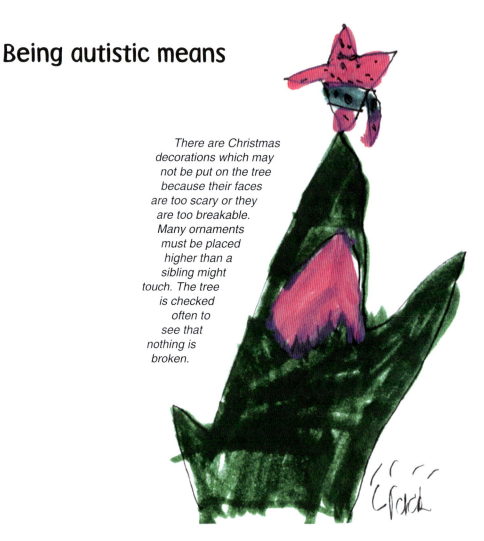

There are Christmas decorations which may not be put on the tree because their faces are too scary or they are too breakable. Many ornaments must be placed higher than a sibling might touch. The tree is checked often to see that nothing is broken.

Target is one of Caspian's most favorite places to go. Unexpectedly, he refused to go one year from mid-October to the first day of December. I found out after he could talk better that Damian had almost touched a Halloween snow globe. The thought of that possibly breaking kept him out of the store until Halloween was over!

Lynne (mother)

He is afraid of any place that has breakables in it. If we are able to get him in the door, we have to make sure no one gets too close to anything fragile.

Parviz (father)

Caspian's cousin Jay is a glass blower. We walked by a broken glass pile on the way into the building to watch Jay work. When Jay wasn't happy with a piece of his artwork, he had Caspian and his brother Damian break the piece in the pile. I had never seen Caspian delight in broken things as he had that day. I think it was a good experience because he was surrounded by love and acceptance and the sound of breaking (tinkling) glass. For a while he seemed less concerned about things breaking.

Jan (aunt)

How about that glass horse. It's in his room but he never lets anyone go near it because he's too afraid.

Damian (brother)

During his kindergarten year, a window at the local fish hatchery had been vandalized. We had to go check it every day after school for weeks to see if it had been repaired.

Lynne (mother)

Caspian was very distressed and almost inconsolable when a page would be ripped in a book. He would have a hard time getting back to the story.

Mrs. N (2nd grade teacher)

Even the sound of mail being opened would set him off.

Lynne (mother)

"The snow globe is broken so I fix it."

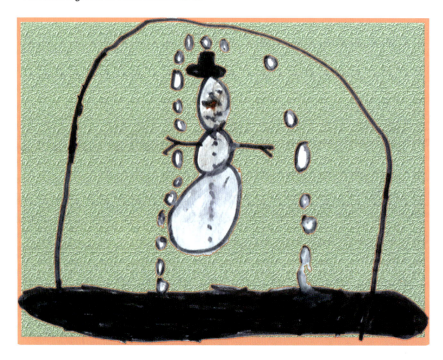

I don't feel safe when things rip or break.

Being autistic means

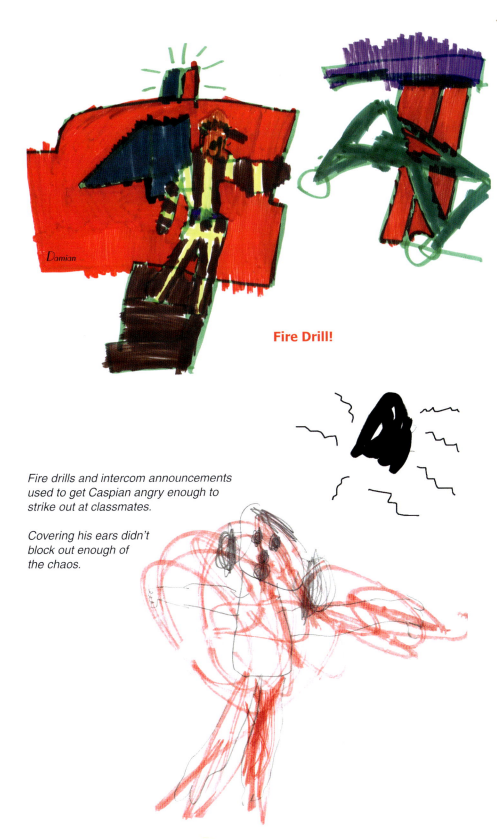

Damian

Fire Drill!

Fire drills and intercom announcements used to get Caspian angry enough to strike out at classmates.

Covering his ears didn't block out enough of the chaos.

when I don't feel safe, I cover my ears. I go away inside myself.

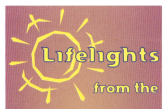
All a stranger had to do was look at Caspian and he would cover his ears. He does this less often now, but still zones when he gets overloaded.
Lynne (mother)

When he overloads, he needs to simplify the world.
Diane (2nd grade EA)

When Caspian doesn't want to listen or do what is asked, he covers his ears and smiles to see if you'll go away.
Ms. H (3rd grade teacher)

Whenever Caspian gets in trouble, he covers his ears.
Rebecca (classmate)

I see him cover his ears in fire drills.
Elise (classmate)

This is how he helps himself feel better.
Anna (2nd & 3rd grade EA)

I have not seen this since 1st grade.
Joy (classroom volunteer)

And sometimes he 'goes away' without any outward sign - except the bleakness in his eyes.
Mina (grandmother)

Caspian learned to take sudden noises more easily during class time when we identified certain noises for him (on purpose) such as the pencil sharpener (which bothered him if it was done at a different time than usual), the chair scraping, dropping staplers, notebooks and pencil boxes. He would still cover his ears and look pained.
Mrs. N (2nd grade teacher)

Caspian covers his ears to eliminate input, not to eliminate sound. Much the same way some people close their eyes when they are trying to follow the harmony in a song.
Lynne (mother)

Being autistic means

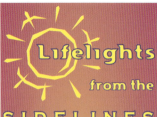

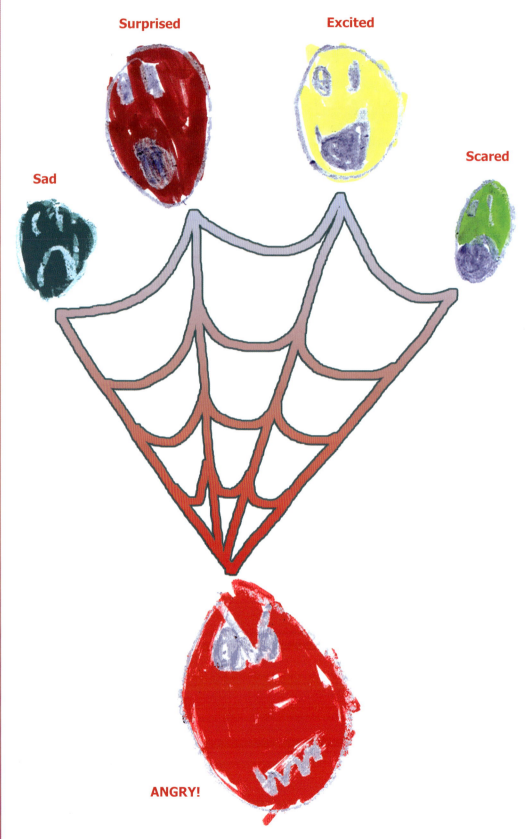

if I can't let my big feelings out they turn into angry feelings fast.

12

How do you react to stress?

Being autistic means

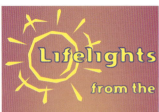

"The happy eyes are scary."

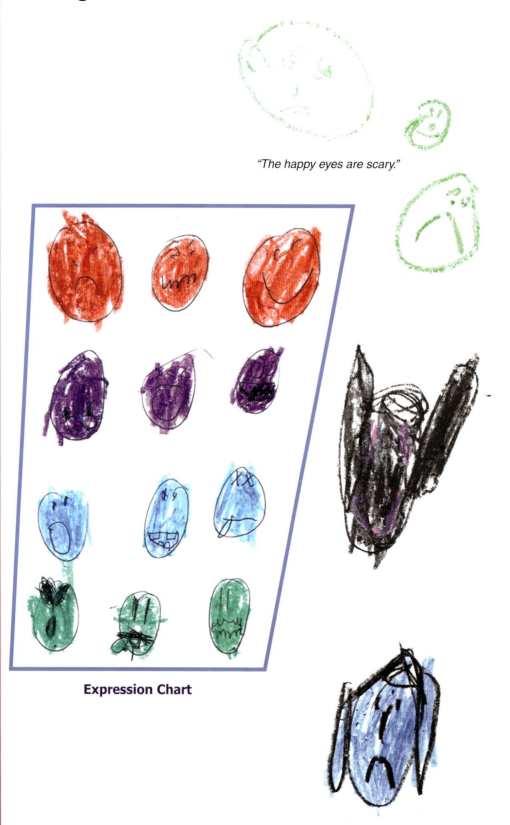

Expression Chart

expressions can confuse me and eyes can scare me. Sometimes happy faces look angry and sad faces look funny.

14

Being autistic means

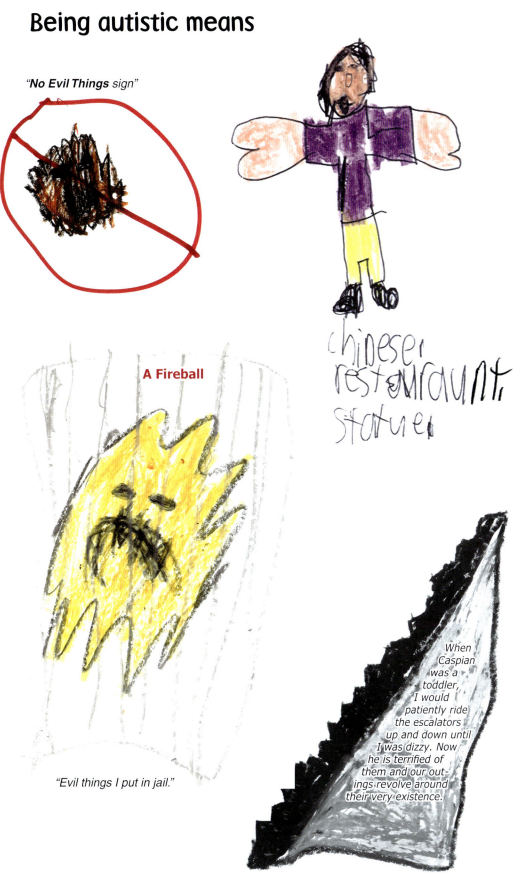

"No Evil Things sign"

A Fireball

"Evil things I put in jail."

chineser restouraunt statue

When Caspian was a toddler, I would patiently ride the escalators up and down until I was dizzy. Now he is terrified of them and our outings revolve around their very existence.

pictures and statues can make me uneasy. I spend a lot of time feeling afraid.

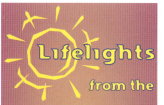
Likenesses of people frighten him much more than photos because he notices that which is not quite right.

Lynne (mother)

This particular fear totally limits our restaurant selection. Malls are out. When we do manage to get him into a mall, there are certain stores we cannot even pass in front of.

Parviz (father)

There used to be a mask hanging on our wall. We took it down 'cause it broke. He asked about it every time he came into our house and showed me where it used to be.

Alejandro (friend)

Caspian didn't like the Grandfather's face in one of our first stories last fall.

Ms. H (3rd grade teacher)

Sometimes he covers up pictures.

Elise (classmate)

I remember when Caspian was young we would choose the restaurants carefully. We always checked for pictures on the wall or statues or stuffed animals. We thought it was the eyes that made him uncomfortable.

Jan (aunt)

They look like people. Are they going to move or talk?

Diane (2nd grade EA)

Like that Indian restaurant. He's afraid of the pictures there. That's why we always have to sit at the table that doesn't have any pictures.

Damian (brother)

I remember one incident where Caspian melted down when a glass of wine was set down for me. He saw his distorted reflection. We had to ditch the glass.

Mina (grandmother)

What frightens you?

Being autistic means

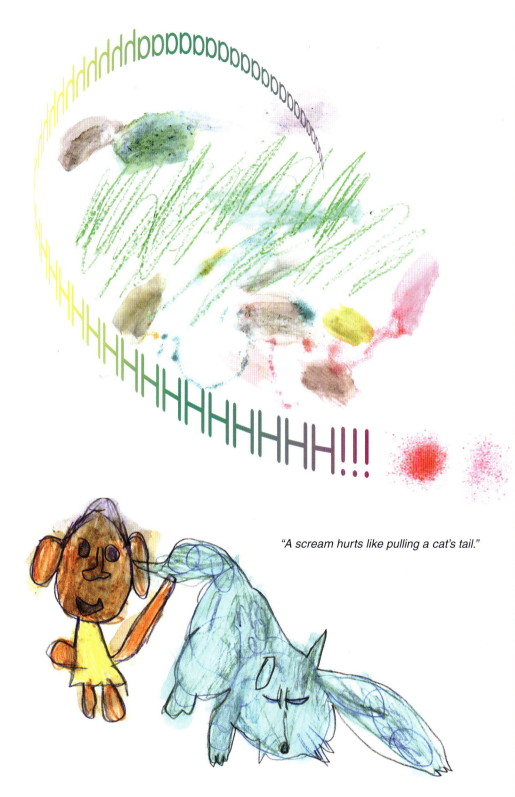

"A scream hurts like pulling a cat's tail."

when people talk loudly or scream, it hurts my ears and hurts my feelings.
Sudden noises confuse me.

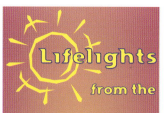

Lifelights from the SIDELINES

Background noise carries as much listening weight as a teacher talking. Unidentifiable sounds or noise patterns can be very scary.

Lynne (mother)

He still won't let me play my music in the house.

Parviz (father)

Caspian likes it when you talk calmly and quietly to him, especially if he's mad. If things get too loud in the classroom, sometimes he will hide under a desk or in a closet. It makes him feel safe until the noise goes away.

Mr. G (1st grade teacher)

Once we were playing outside and somebody started mowing the grass. He got scared so we had to go somewhere else.

Alejandro (friend)

When people talk loudly he asks, "Are you angry?"

Ms. H (3rd grade teacher)

In a fire drill he sometimes walks around the room in confusion.

Elise (classmate)

The 5th grade would walk past us quite often while reading out in the hall. There were many loud noises. Caspian concentrated as well or better than other 3rd graders.

Joy (classroom volunteer)

Sound is intense. He hears things louder than we do.

Diane (2nd grade EA)

Atesha screamed for Mommy and Caspian yelled at Atesha for screaming.

Damian (brother)

To get back at someone, he sometimes says *shhhh* to them. This is because this sound is painful to his own ears. When he was learning to read, he would not read words that started with the letter M. Sounding out slowly made the *mmmm* sound vibrate in his stomach uncomfortably.

Lynne (mother)

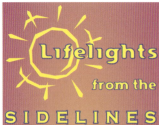

Being autistic means

When I try to sit with my arm around him, he pulls back.
Parviz (father)

When we want to show a child our love and affection we give them a hug, kiss or even tousle their hair and tell them we love them. To hug Caspian you must first ask him if he'll let you give him a hug. If he says it's okay to hug him it will be better for him if it's a quick hug. Physical contact can be uncomfortable to him. What bothers me most about this is I don't think he understands how much we love him.
Cindy (aunt)

When Caspian is upset, he doesn't like it when people hover around him. He needs some time and some space.
Mr. G (1st grade teacher)

I know that when I get a migraine, light seems so bright I want to shut my eyes. Smell becomes so intense it makes me nauseous and touch hurts like I'm covered in burns. I wonder if he feels similar?
Diane (2nd grade EA)

Sometimes when we are playing rough with Damian he gets mad fast.
Alejandro (friend)

He sits away at group time on the rug to avoid being close to others.
Ms. H (3rd grade teacher)

Sometimes when I touch him he glares at me.
Elise (classmate)

I've learned to say when I'm going to touch him to fix a technique *before* I do it. Sometimes when I touch him, he will touch himself in the same spot like he is wiping it off.
Jennifer (martial arts instructor)

His skin is very sensitive. When he was little, he would make me draw and write on his back and he'd try to guess what I was drawing. Yet even with such sensitivity, he has a high pain tolerance. If someone taps him on the shoulder to ask his name, he reacts as if he's been hit. But if he falls from a high stool to the ground, he simply states, "I'm upside-down!"
Lynne (mother)

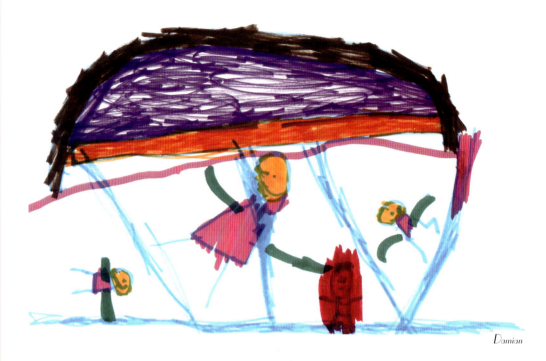

Damian

"My friend tags me, so I am making an angry face."

Even a drop of water on his clothing evokes a pained reaction

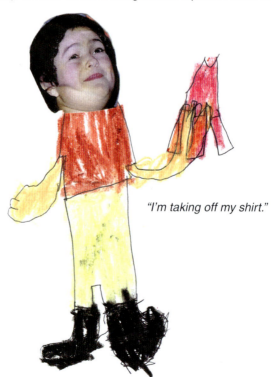

"I'm taking off my shirt."

sometimes when someone touches me, it hurts like they are hitting me instead.

18

Being autistic means

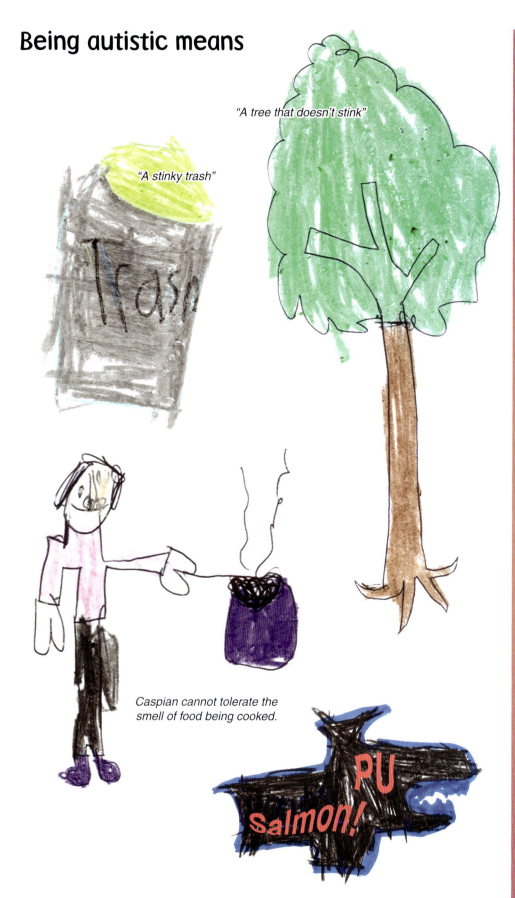

"A tree that doesn't stink"

"A stinky trash"

Caspian cannot tolerate the smell of food being cooked.

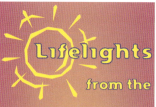
We started naming foods after his favorite film characters to get him to try new things (everything smelled bad to him). Snoopy sandwich, Ewok salad, Jafar apples, etc.

Lynne (mother)

He can't stand it when I cook food, he won't try new foods, he won't even come to the table and he won't let anyone with a bowl of cooked food sit in the same room with him.

Parviz (father)

Caspian backs up quickly on the rug if another student passes gas.

Ms. H (3rd grade teacher)

Smells are too intense. Even a good thing can seem bad when it's too much.

Diane (2nd grade EA)

He doesn't like the way your food smells.

Damian (brother)

Caspian refused to go into the ice cream parlor in town. He would cover his ears and stare at a picture of steam over a bowl of soup and then run out. After he could talk better, I learned that it was not the picture, but the smell of the owner's lunch that kept him from entering the first time. Subsequent times it was the memory of the smell that kept him out.

Lynne (mother)

Caspian would often tell me he didn't like the smell of something by the way he acted rather than with words. He would make a very strong displeased facial expression and make noises.

Mrs. N (2nd grade teacher)

I don't like the way things smell. It makes me want to run away!

What bothers you?

Being autistic means

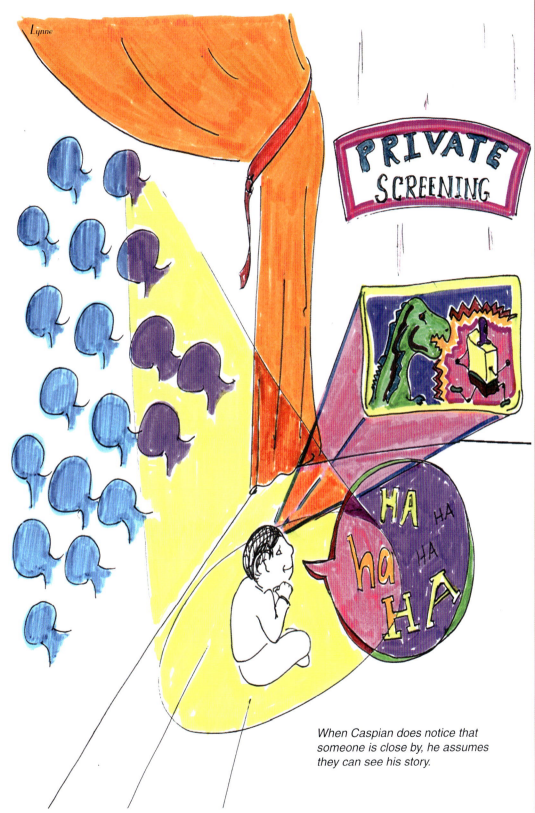

Lynne

PRIVATE SCREENING

When Caspian does notice that someone is close by, he assumes they can see his story.

I say things out loud or act out stories to myself. I don't always know that others can hear me.

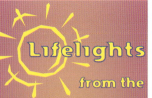

Lifelights from the SIDELINES

I'm so used to this I don't even hear it anymore. But I'll never forget when his vacant repetition started turning into real comments!

Lynne (mother)

I notice this mostly when we're watching TV together in the evenings. He spends most of his time repeating other stories and not watching what's on.

Parviz (father)

He says some things when we are playing. Like he talks in a whisper. I used to do that too when I pretended to announce my own moves when I played soccer.

Alejandro (friend)

Just the other day Caspian was voicing each word as he was writing it even after another student asked him to stop. He was oblivious to the other students.

Ms. H (3rd grade teacher)

Sometimes in the middle of quiet time Caspian will yell out something. He surprises us!

Rebecca (classmate)

He always pretends to turn the class into frogs!

Elise (classmate)

His mind is very creative. He enjoys making stories.

Anna (2nd & 3rd grade EA)

I've heard him say out loud what he thinks of other children's behavior as he watches class - he seems not to realize they will hear what he is saying.

Laurel (martial arts instructor)

When he's in his special world he's focused on the inside and the outside gets lost.

Diane (2nd grade EA)

I have heard Caspian repeat entire scenes from a movie and Lynne says that it was verbatim.

Mina (grandmother)

Being autistic means

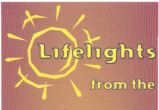
I tell his teachers that when he is told something in the presence of more than one person, it should be assumed that he didn't hear any of it.

Lynne (mother)

At times when I want to get his attention it's pretty hard. And then to keep his attention is still a challenge.

Parviz (father)

Sometimes when me and Damian are making teams we call him to play with us but he keeps not answering.

Alejandro (friend)

Caspian responds with, "Ya?" after you call his name

Ms. H (3rd grade teacher)

Sometimes when I am looking at him he seems to be staring at something funny.

Elise (classmate)

I know, it takes me like 10 times for me to get his attention.

Damian (brother)

Call my name first is right. And, sometimes, make sure that you have eye contact.

Mina (grandmother)

Caspian preferred to be in his own world most of the time, thinking his own stories and 'playing' with his friends simply by knowing they were in the vicinity. It took a lot of time and effort to draw him out of his thinking and into the world around him. Sometimes he would tune in for a few minutes; sometimes for just a split second - but long enough for me to find the pattern of words that got his attention. His desire to interact with others has been his saving grace. Nowadays he spends more time engaged than not. There was a time when I feared that would never happen.

Lynne (mother)

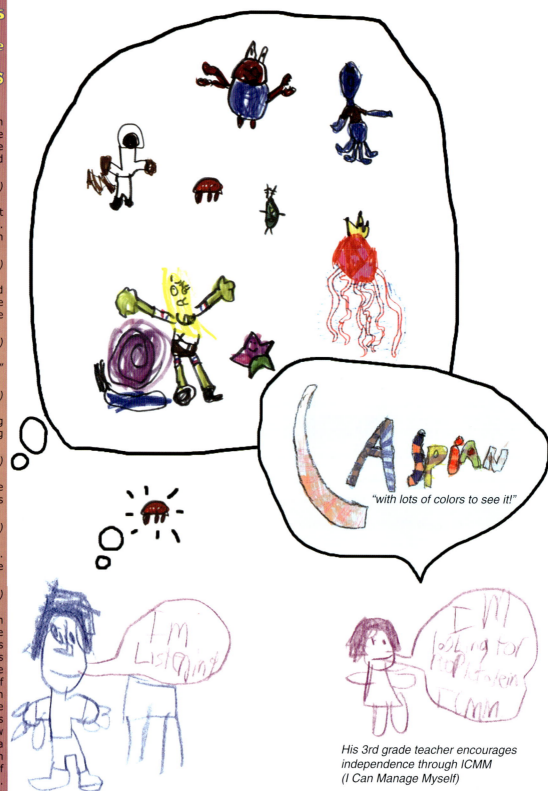

"with lots of colors to see it!"

His 3rd grade teacher encourages independence through ICMM (I Can Manage Myself)

when I'm thinking about my own stories, it's hard for me to hear you. If you want to tell me something, call my name first.

22

Being autistic means

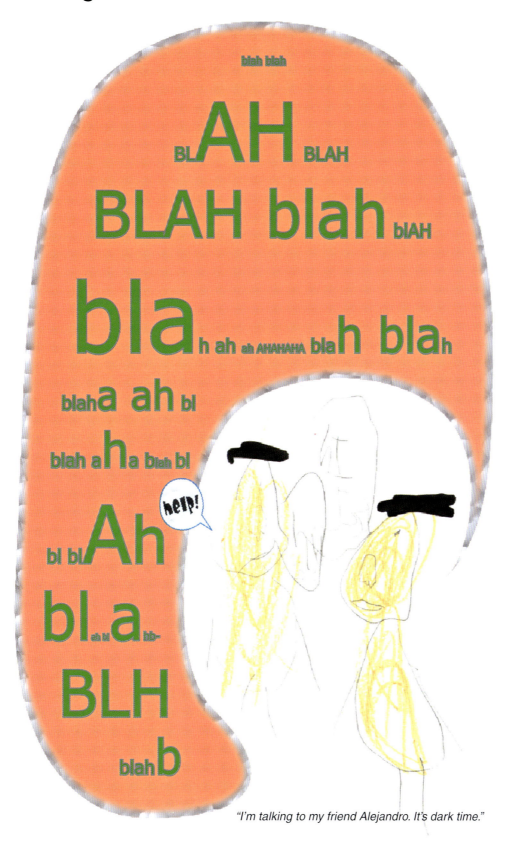

"I'm talking to my friend Alejandro. It's dark time."

I don't always know how loudly I am talking or how close to someone I am standing.

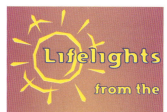

I used to be so glad he was talking that I didn't care how loudly he was doing it! But I've seen the look on his classmates' faces when he practically pins them to the wall telling an exciting story loudly into their faces.

Lynne (mother)

I don't notice how loud he talks until I need him to be quiet so he won't wake his sister.

Parviz (father)

Sometimes Caspian says, "I don't like you!" But he really doesn't mean it. He is just angry.

Mr. G (1st grade teacher)

Personal space is learned. Some people never quite get it!

Diane (2nd grade EA)

When he's standing near me he gets too close.

Alejandro (friend)

He needs constant reminders and visual cues to use a quiet voice.

Ms. H (3rd grade teacher)

A reminder to 'turn the volume down' or give personal space is fine.

Anna (2nd & 3rd grade EA)

I love the way Caspian looks at me and says, "Hi!" when I say hello to him.

Joy (classroom volunteer)

'Cause sometimes he goes back to dreaming in the middle of a sentence.

Damian (brother)

At times Caspian would get angry when shushed by the teacher. He would exaggeratedly make the same sounds over and over (and then smile or frown). He would respond to my facial expressions.

Mrs. N (2nd grade teacher)

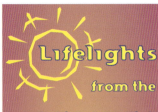
Caspian started out in a bilingual household. He was making the same mistakes in both languages; he did not know when one word ended and another began. I started really slowing my speech down. I could tell by the tilt of his head that he understood a little more.

Lynne (mother)

Whenever I ask him for details about his day he tells me he is too tired to talk about it.

Parviz (father)

Sometimes Caspian will begin talking to you about something that happened to him a long time ago just like it was yesterday. He doesn't realize how much time has passed.

Mr. G (1st grade teacher)

He works hard in his brain to think of replies and information. If it gets too hard he says, "I don't know." Sometimes he gets angry when he doesn't know the answers.

Anna (2nd & 3rd grade EA)

Caspian will often repeat phrases up to the point where retrieval is missing. He eventually expresses his idea after describing it in different words.

Ms. H (3rd grade teacher)

His head is full of soooo much information! It's hard to break it down - make it simple.

Diane (2nd grade EA)

When searching for a way to communicate, Caspian would say whatever he most remembered from that same situation. He would say, "Are you OK?" if he got hurt. "Then we have a picnic at Cherry Creek Park" became the name of a nearby grocery store because that's what I had said to him in the parking lot. A Diet Coke was called "Give it to Joe!" because that's what was said to him the last time one was in his hand.

Lynne (mother)

Being autistic means

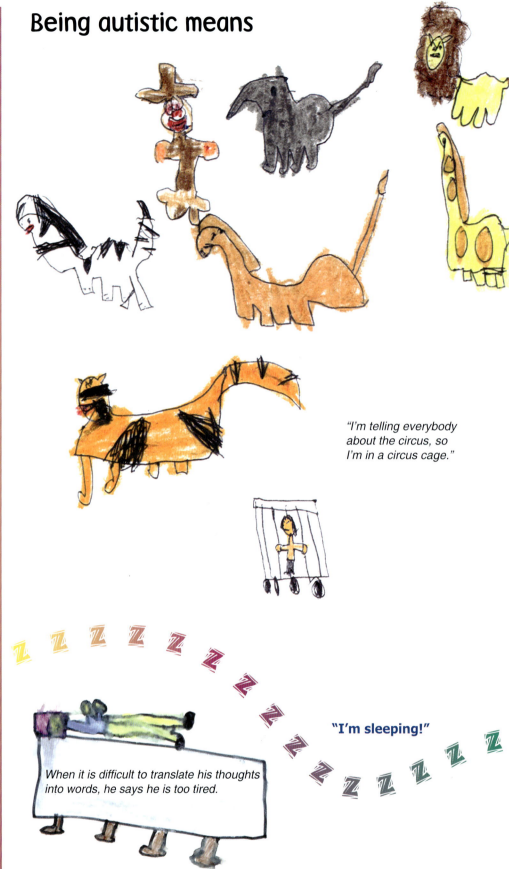

"I'm telling everybody about the circus, so I'm in a circus cage."

"I'm sleeping!"

When it is difficult to translate his thoughts into words, he says he is too tired.

it's hard for me to find the words I need to answer questions or tell stories.

24

Being autistic means

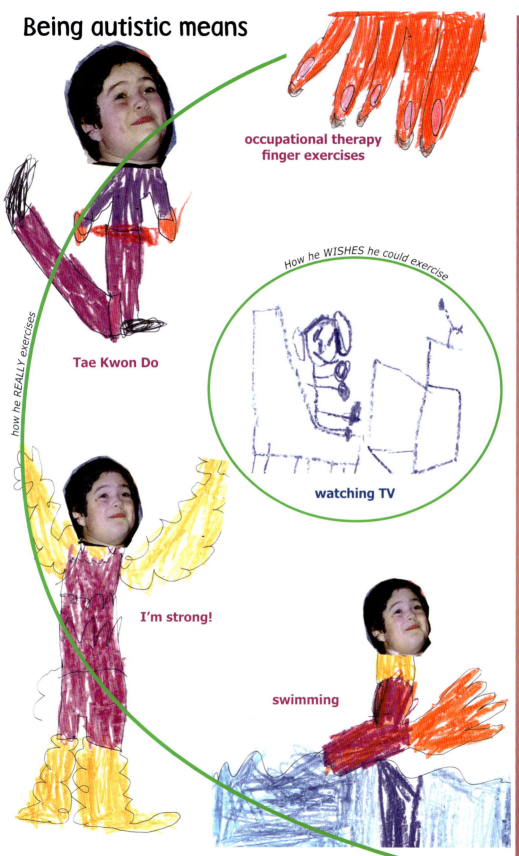

occupational therapy
finger exercises

How he WISHES he could exercise

how he REALLY exercises

Tae Kwon Do

watching TV

I'm strong!

swimming

I have to work very hard to make my
muscles strong - even the little ones in
my fingers!

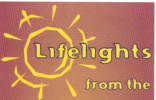
It's not easy to keep him active.

Parviz (father)

He is getting stronger because we help each other with hand weights.

Alejandro (friend)

He enjoys games in PE. Sometimes they are difficult for him but he does what he can. He gets frustrated during team games a lot because they can be too fast

Anna (2nd & 3rd grade EA)

Jumping rope might seem simple, but it's jumping at the perfect time while making his arms make the rope swing around his body while 'seeing' the movement of the rope. Lots going on!

Diane (2nd grade EA)

Like when he gets excited he looks kind of funny the way he moves his body.

Damian (brother)

Caspian gets tired after just a little exercise. He's learned to say so without using the 't' word, though, because then we do pushups (one may not say the word 'tired' on the training floor).

We work on strength and flexibility in every class. Most kids Caspian's age are really limber and hardly need to stretch, but Caspian has to work at it.

We set goals ("count to ten in Korean", "count to twenty in Spanish") to make exercise and stretch fun and to make sure we do enough.

Jennifer (martial arts instructor)

Keeping him in engaged in regular physical activity is furiously difficult and desperately important. As a toddler, swimming increased his speech; but it was hard to find a quiet pool!

Lynne (mother)

Writing with frames helped Caspian to determine size in 2nd grade.

Mrs. N (2nd grade teacher)

25

Being autistic means

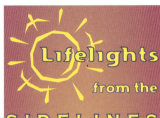

This makes him very genuine, since he never tries to tailor his answer to his audience. It can also make him appear impolite for the same reason.

Lynne (mother)

He knows when *he's* hurts. He knows when *he's* happy.

Diane (2nd grade EA)

He often says, "You mean..." and waits for an explanation to fit into his own frame of reference.

Ms. H (3rd grade teacher)

He doesn't always know when you're upset with him. Sometimes he asks if you are angry because he's not sure about the expression on your face.

Anna (2nd & 3rd grade EA)

If you see the world from your point of view - that's what counts. No one knows what others are feeling.

Joy (classroom volunteer)

Caspian can't even guess. He needs to be taught how facial expressions relate to emotion. Even his own 'angry face' is practiced, and, well, still cute to me. The biggest breakthrough we had in understanding expressions involved a little camera connected to the computer. He would make faces into the camera, record little movies of himself and take snapshots of different expressions.

Lynne (mother)

Caspian would sometimes strike out when he misunderstood the signals of others. It took some time before he could hear that they were not meaning what he thought. He would repeat the teacher's message many times to make it clear in his own mind and to keep himself from reacting.

Mrs. N (2nd grade teacher)

He will try to bite his sibling's fingernails when they are long because it bothers him when his own are long. He also presses on Atesha's bellybutton because it must feel good to her, too!

Lynne (mother)

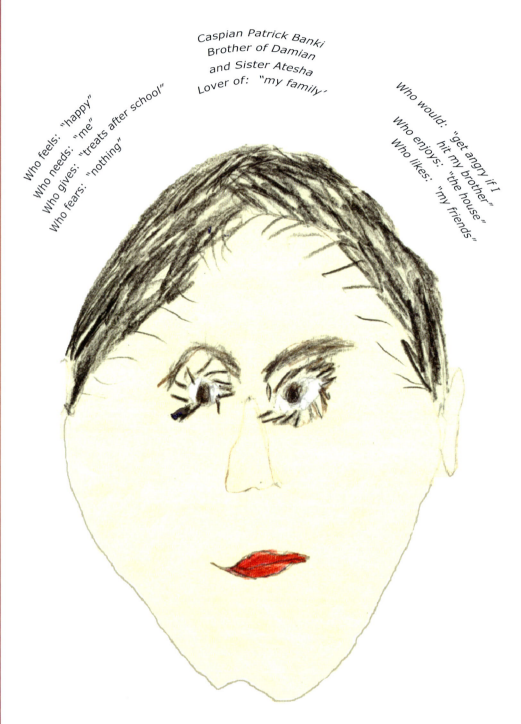

Caspian Patrick Banki
Brother of Damian
and Sister Atesha
Lover of: "my family"

Who feels: "happy"
Who needs: "me"
Who gives: "treats after school"
Who fears: "nothing"

Who would: "get angry if I hit my brother"
Who enjoys: "the house"
Who likes: "my friends"

I see the world from my point of view first and it is difficult for me to guess what others are feeling.

What challenges you?

Being autistic means

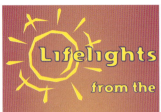

Damian was the first child to fully comprehend Caspian's method of play. He is still Caspian's best teacher.

Lynne (mother)

Caspian likes to feel proud of himself just like other kids. He likes it when you say nice things to him.

Mr. G (1st grade teacher)

Once me, Caspian and Damian were playing with worms. Caspian didn't want to touch the worms. So he held the cup for us.

Alejandro (friend)

Caspian responds positively when approached with, "I need your help."

Ms. H (3rd grade teacher)

Not everyone plays by the rules. Sometimes people are aggressive - this makes him respond with the same.

Diane (2nd grade EA)

What is "normal"? Are allergies "normal"? Is wearing glasses "normal"? We consider all these things "normal" because they are common. If everyone knew a child with autism that would be "normal" too.

Cindy (aunt)

This is difficult because Caspian gets angry at kids when they correct him, like it's criticism not assistance.

Anna (2nd & 3rd grade EA)

Just a week or so ago we did full body outlines. I was so pleased when I stepped back into the classroom to get another two children to take turns doing each other's outline. Caspian had his hand up and asked if he could 'please be next' he and Ben. When Caspian laid out on the paper he mentioned that he was 'born different and had a hard time holding still'. As it was he *did* hold as still as everyone else!

Joy (classroom volunteer)

Lynne, he's going to be just fine.

Nee (great-grandmother)

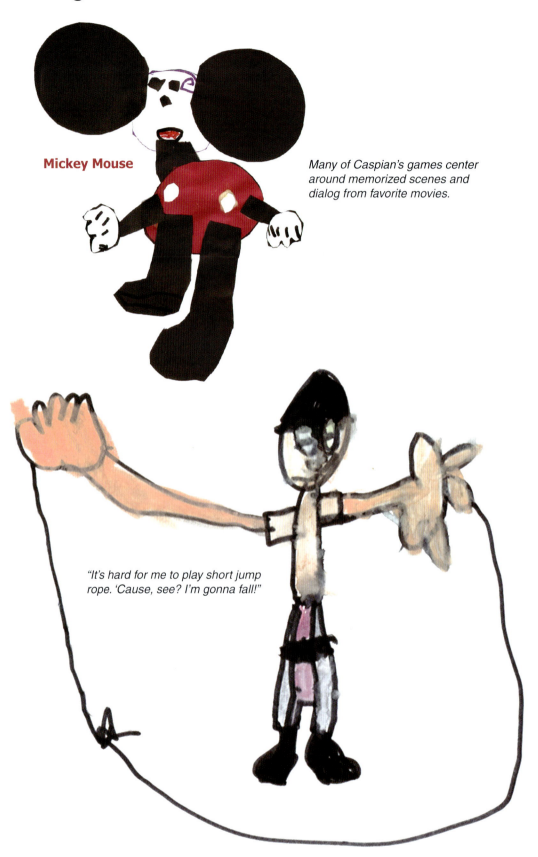

Mickey Mouse

Many of Caspian's games center around memorized scenes and dialog from favorite movies.

"It's hard for me to play short jump rope. 'Cause, see? I'm gonna fall!"

sometimes it's hard for us to understand each other's games. Let's teach each other!

I was born with autism. That makes me different. What makes you different?

What makes you different?

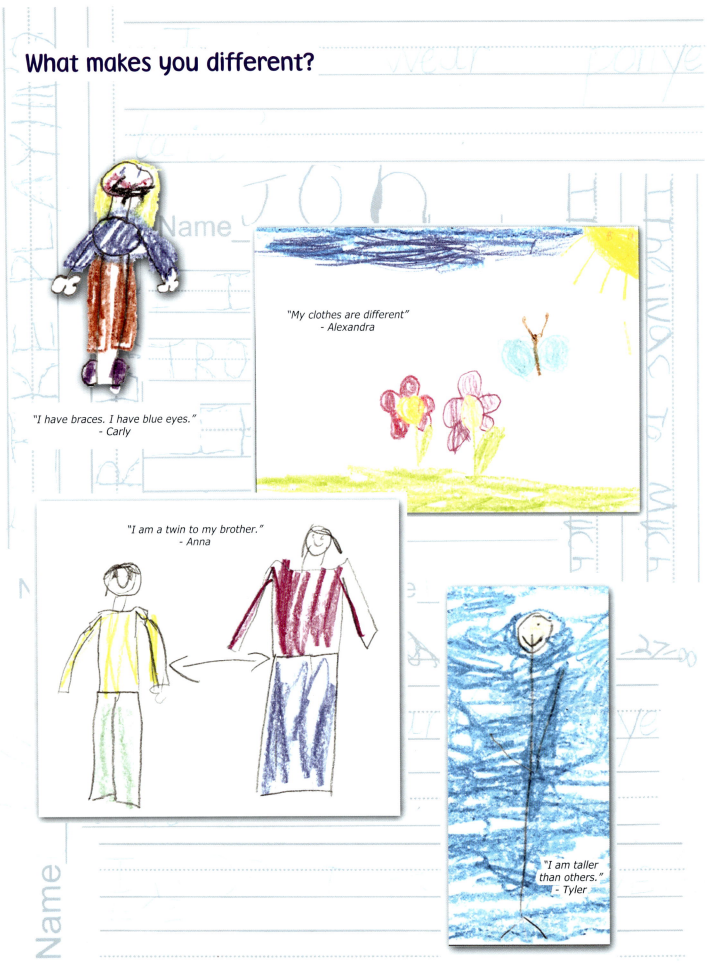

"I have braces. I have blue eyes."
- Carly

"My clothes are different"
- Alexandra

"I am a twin to my brother."
- Anna

"I am taller than others."
- Tyler

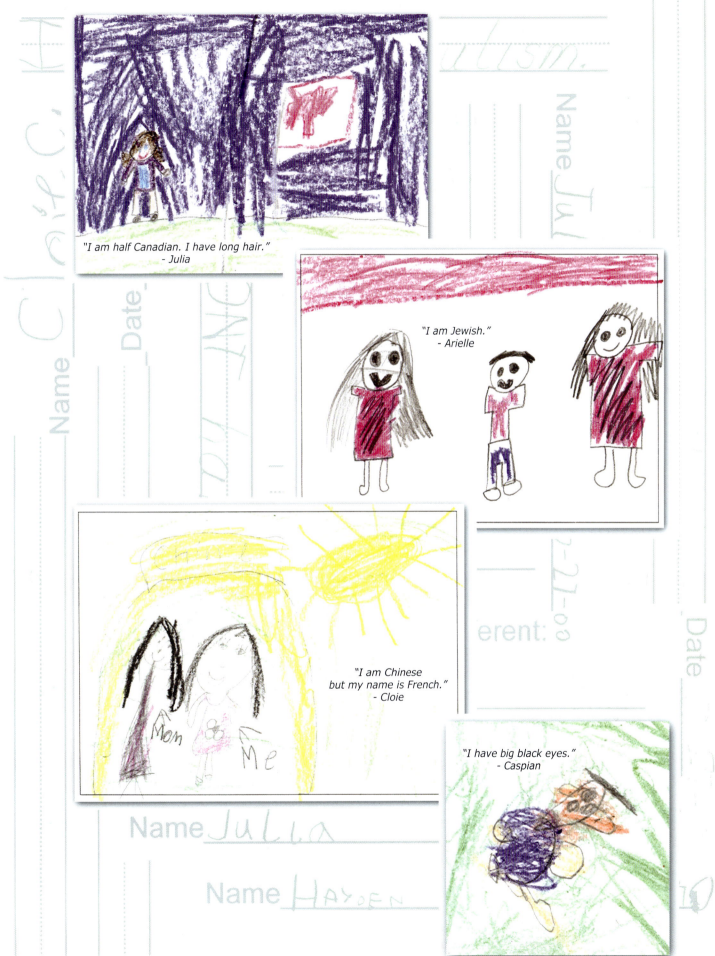

"I am half Canadian. I have long hair."
- Julia

"I am Jewish."
- Arielle

"I am Chinese
but my name is French."
- Cloie

"I have big black eyes."
- Caspian

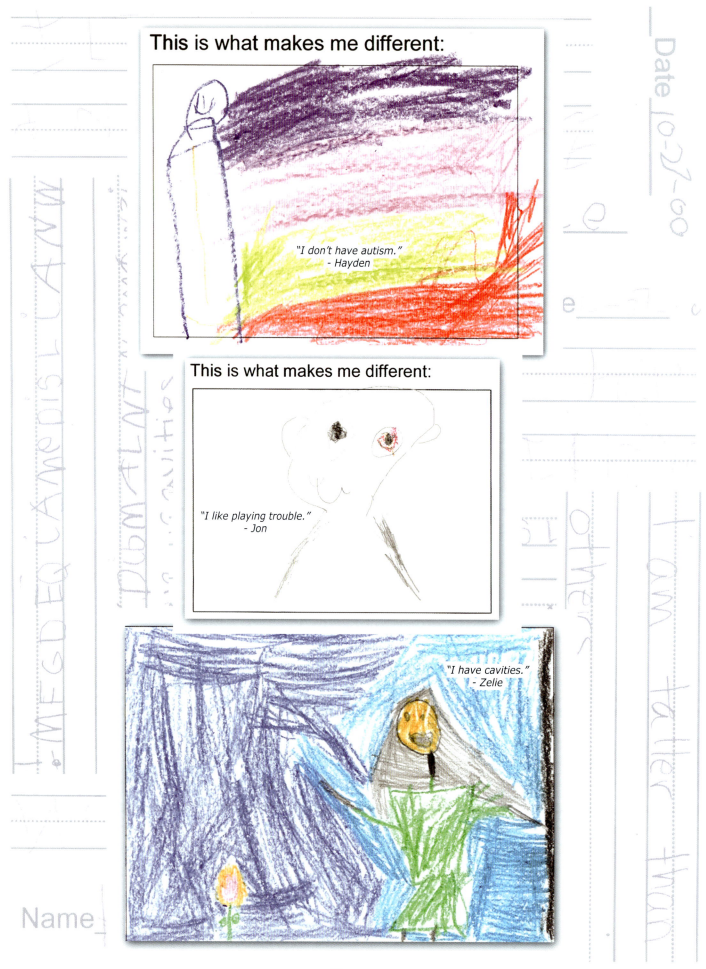

This is what makes me different:

"I don't have autism."
- Hayden

This is what makes me different:

"I like playing trouble."
- Jon

"I have cavities."
- Zelie

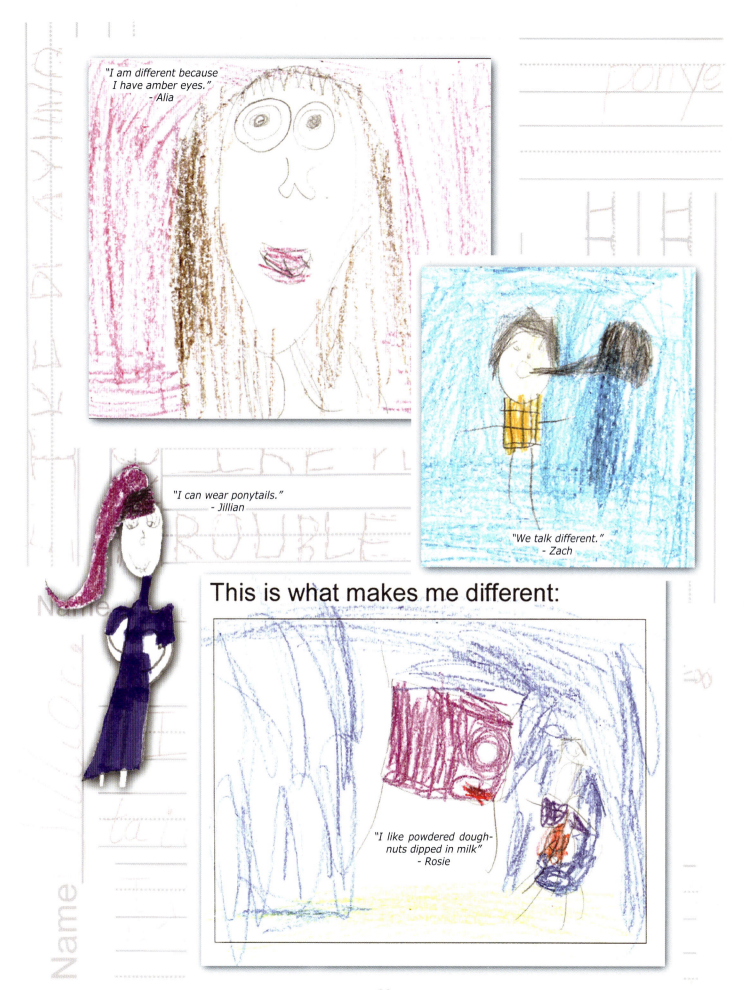

*"I am different because
I have amber eyes."*
- Alia

"I can wear ponytails."
- Jillian

"We talk different."
- Zach

This is what makes me different:

*"I like powdered dough-
nuts dipped in milk"*
- Rosie

Autistic children are all different. Being Caspian's aunt in no way makes me an expert on autism. What I have learned from Caspian is that we must not judge and assume. I no longer look at the tantruming child in the grocery store with a judging eye. Each child is motivated by thoughts and feelings far beyond our understanding. I have watched Caspian's mother work tirelessly over the years to give Caspian the language skills that make him capable of telling his mother what motivates his 'odd' behaviors. Once understood, his behaviors make far more sense. I have watched Caspian's mother handle an overwhelmed and distraught child with such calm, only to have it all thrown away by the comment of a stranger who feels that his input of, 'listen to your mother, son' is going to fix the situation.

This book celebrates uniqueness, but there is one thing that all people share. When others are mean to us, it hurts our feelings. Sometimes people are mean because they don't understand the motivations behind the behaviors they observe. Everyone has had his or her feelings hurt by someone else. Children like Caspian, and parents like my sister, have been hurt over and over again by people who have no understanding of the miracle of Caspian.

Caspian's miracle is that he speaks his own words in his own voice, even if that voice is sometimes a bit too obsessively insistent (yet still polite) that he needs to use the phone 'now' to call a friend (yes, you read that right - using a *telephone* and calling a *friend*). Caspian's miracle is that he hugs his sister, even if sometimes he hugs her so much she cries. Caspian's miracle is that he had a mother who heard his voice before he could find it, and led him to a place where he now has the voice to speak and the power to express his feelings. If people could see the miracle, they may not be so quick to judge what they don't understand.

Caspian has autism; it is a part of him. He accepts it much the same way a child accepts that he has blue eyes or red hair. It is simply a fact. We don't whisper about the color of people's hair or eyes, we simply accept it as a part of what makes that person unique.

This book is a great tool for parents of autistic children entering grade school, but it is so much more. This book can help parents and grandparents of young autistic children to understand some of the mysterious behaviors of their own children. It can be used as a tool in colleges and schools to educate teachers and students. It is a stepping-stone to understanding some of the motivations behind autistic behavior.

It is a tribute to both Caspian and his mother that this book was ever written. It is a tribute to their strength and endurance that Caspian was in a regular Ed setting in first grade and there was even a need for this book to be written. This book is the miracle of a young autistic boy who has found the voice that many people with autism are still searching for.

Patricia Byrne (Caspian's aunt)